Let Your True Beauty Shine

Over 30 Nourishing, Exfoliating
and Hydrating Facial Scrub
Recipes

BY

Jenny Kings

License Notes

No part of this Book can be reproduced in any form or by any means including print, electronic, scanning or photocopying unless prior permission is granted by the author.

All ideas, suggestions and guidelines mentioned here are written for informative purposes. While the author has taken every possible step to ensure accuracy, all readers are advised to follow information at their own risk. The author cannot be held responsible for personal and/or commercial damages in case of misinterpreting and misunderstanding any part of this Book

Table of Contents

Homemade Facial Scrub Recipes

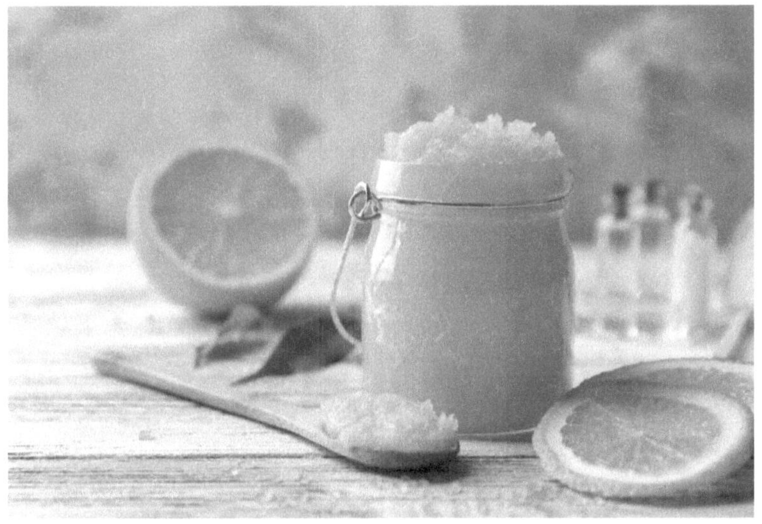

OOOOOOOOOOOOOOOOOOOOOOOOOOOOOOOOOOOOOO

Chapter I - For Dull Skin

OOOOOOOOOOOOOOOOOOOOOOOOOOOOOOOOOOOOOOOO

(1) Turmeric Scrub

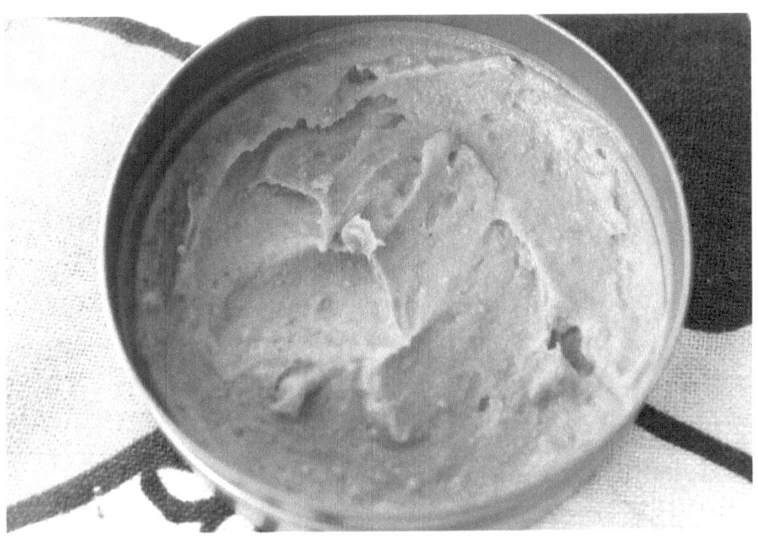

A mild scrub for dry and normal skin types. To cleanse, clarify, and whiten the complexion. Turmeric and milk have skin-whitening compounds that can naturally enhance the color of your skin tone.

Preparation Time: 30 mins

List of Ingredients:

- 1 tablespoon rice powder
- 2 tablespoons gram powder
- ½ teaspoons turmeric
- Small amount of milk

OOOOOOOOOOOOOOOOOOOOOOOOOOOOOOOOOOOOOOO

Procedure:

1. In a small, clean bowl combine all five ingredients and, using a spoon, mix to form a paste.

2. Ensuring that your face is makeup-free, moisten your face, neck, and decolletage with water and lightly scrub the paste into your skin for 2-3 minutes in circular motions.

3. Leave the scrub for 15-20 minutes before rinsing off with warm water. Pat dry with a clean towel. Do not rub.

(2) Kiwi Glow Scrub

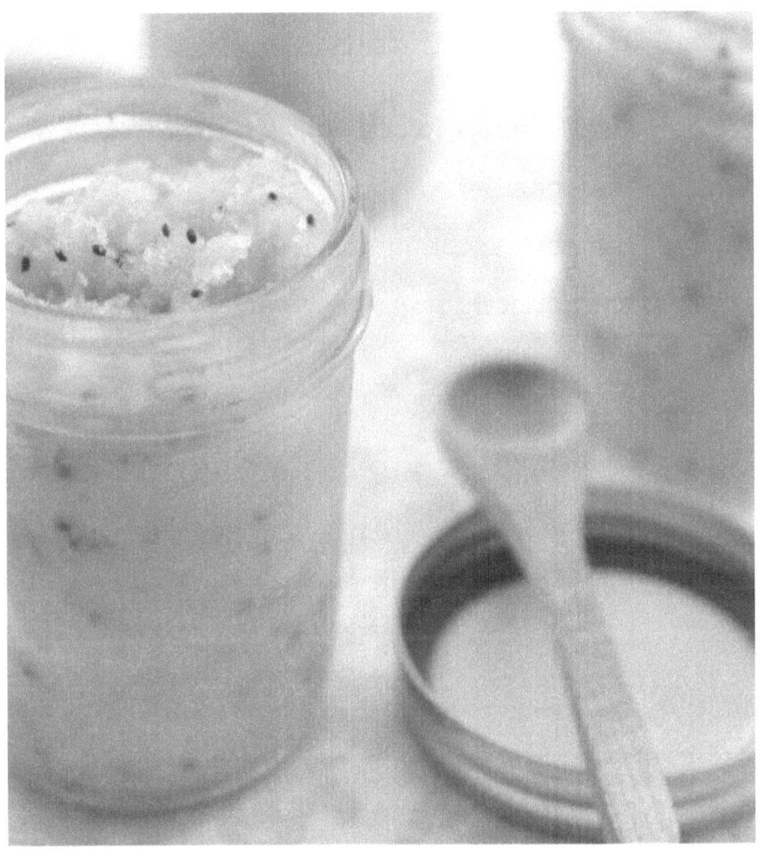

Kiwi contains powerful enzymes. They will work on your skin immediately, removing built-up dead skin cells to reveal a brighter, smoother, and softer complexion. This mask is great for oily skin as the recipe only calls for a small amount of oil.

Preparation Time: 10 mins

List of Ingredients:

- 1 ripe, fresh kiwi
- ½ fresh lemon, juiced
- 1 teaspoon honey
- 1 teaspoon coconut oil
- 3 teaspoons light brown sugar

OOOOOOOOOOOOOOOOOOOOOOOOOOOOOOOOOOOOOOO

Procedure:

1. Peel your kiwi and add it to a blender with all the other ingredients. Blitz the mixture until smooth. Transfer to a small bowl and stir in the sugar until well combined.

2. First, rinse your face with warm water and apply a tablespoon of the mixture to your face, using small, circular motions. Massage into the skin for 2-3 minutes. Wash the mask off using warm water, followed by cold water to re-close your pores.

3. Store any remaining scrub in a jar in the refrigerator*.

*Kiwi scrub will last for 5-7 days in a refrigerator. Use no more than twice a week.

(3) Summer Glow Papaya Scrub

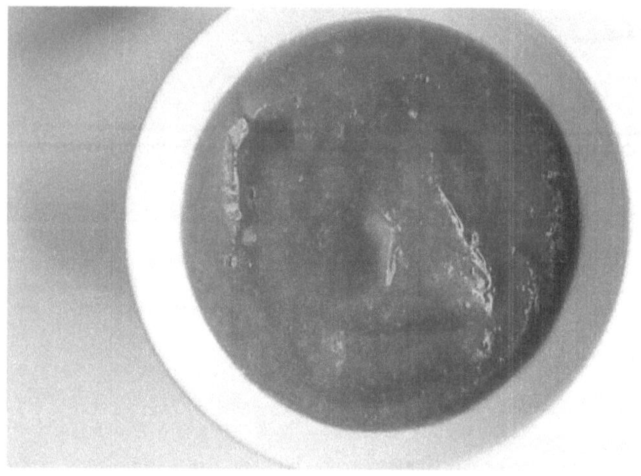

This scrub is ideal for summer, not only will it give you a beautiful, sunshiny glow, but it will soothe sun-damaged skin and naturally lighten sun tans. Use this 2-3 times a week for one month for beautiful summer skin your friends will be jealous of.

Preparation Time: 20 mins

List of Ingredients:

- 2 slices fresh, ripe papaya
- 2 teaspoons honey
- 2 tablespoons whole-fat yogurt
- ½ fresh lemon, juiced
- 2 tablespoons rosewater
- 2 tablespoons light brown sugar

OOOOOOOOOOOOOOOOOOOOOOOOOOOOOOOOOOOOOOO

Procedure:

1. Combine all ingredients in a small bowl and stir well with a spoon*.

2. Apply the scrub to your face and neck. Allow to set for 15-20 minutes before rinsing away with warm water, followed by cold water to re-close your pores.

3. Pat your face dry with a soft towel.

*If you're using this scrub to treat sunburnt skin, place the scrub in the refrigerator for 20 minutes before use for an extra-soothing effect.

(4) Apple and Oatmeal Scrub

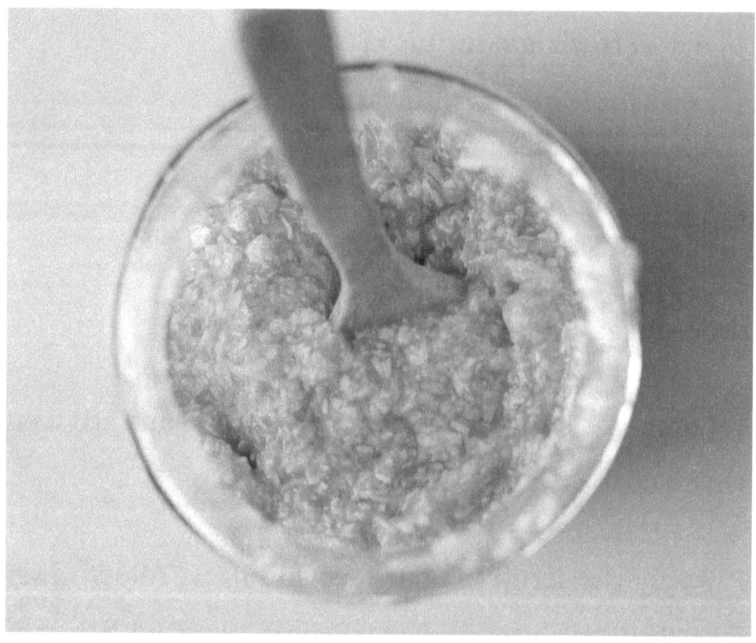

Oatmeal is not just for breakfast! It is an excellent way to exfoliate the skin and, combined with apple and honey, you will have a complexion that is supple and glowing all day.

Preparation Time: 10 mins

List of Ingredients:

- ½ fresh apple
- 1 tablespoon oatmeal
- 1 tablespoon cornmeal
- 1 teaspoon organic honey (optional)

ooooooooooooooooooooooooooooooooooooooooo

Procedure:

1. First, prepare your skin by washing in warm water and patting dry.

2. In a blender, add the apple, oatmeal, and cornmeal. Blend well to form a paste. If the apple does not have sufficient juice to form a paste simply add a little honey.

3. Apply to the face with clean, moist fingertips in circular movements. Massage gently into the skin for 2-3 minutes.

4. Rinse off with warm water using a cotton pad or wet cloth, and pat dry with a clean towel. Do not rub.

5. Apply moisturizer to the skin.

(5) Tropical Papaya and Pineapple Scrub

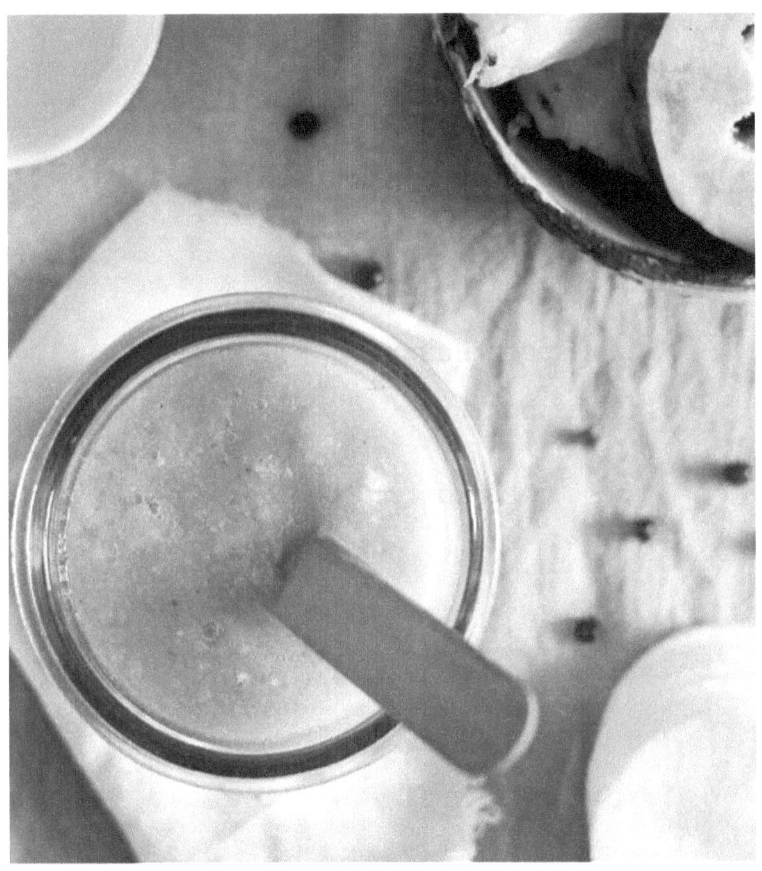

You'll have to remind yourself not to eat this deliciously tropical-smelling scrub! Together, pineapple and papaya contain bromelain and vitamin

A; both of which help to get rid of dead skin cells and inflammation that can lead to a dull, lifeless-looking complexion. Use once a week for bright, glowing skin.

Preparation Time: 10 mins

List of Ingredients:

- ¼ cup fresh pineapple, cubed
- ¼ cup fresh papaya, cubed
- 2 tablespoons light brown sugar
- 1 tablespoon almond oil
- 1 tablespoon honey

OOOOOOOOOOOOOOOOOOOOOOOOOOOOOOOOOOOOOOO

Procedure:

1. Puree the pineapple and papaya in a food processor. Transfer to a small bowl.

2. Add in the remaining ingredients and stir until well combined. Apply the scrub to your clean, dry face. Allow the scrub to sit for a few minutes.

3. Use circular motions and warm water to rinse the scrub from your face. Pat your skin dry with a soft towel.

(6) Berry Granola Scrub

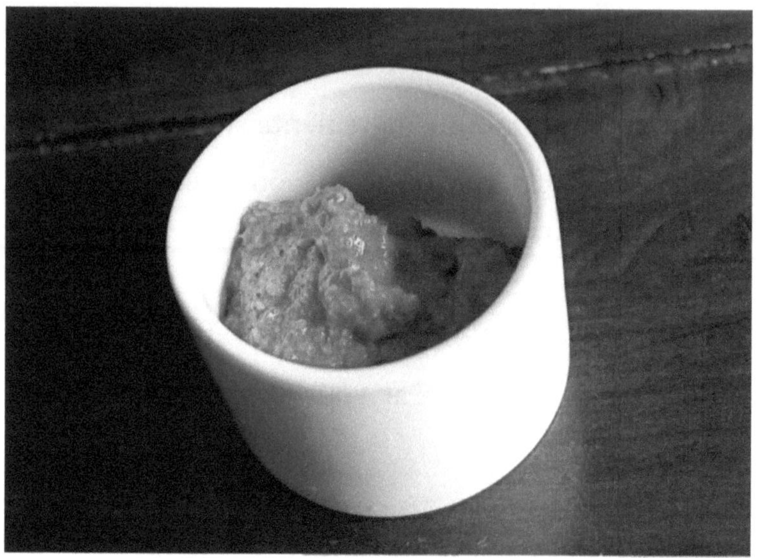

Raw almonds and antioxidant-rich blueberries are chock-full of vitamin E and fatty acids. With anti-inflammatory oats and brightening milk and honey, this scrub is better than any chemical-packed mixture you would find in a store.

Preparation Time: 30 mins

List of Ingredients:

- ½ cup fresh blueberries
- ¼ cup raw almonds
- 2 tablespoons rolled oats
- 1 tablespoon runny honey
- 1 tablespoon organic, whole milk

OOOOOOOOOOOOOOOOOOOOOOOOOOOOOOOOOOOOOOOO

Procedure:

1. Combine all the ingredients in a blender and blitz until smooth.

2. Apply the scrub to your skin and allow to sit and harden for 15-20 minutes.

3. Wet your hands with cold water and massage the scrub into your skin using gentle, circular motions for 1-2 minutes.

4. Rinse the scrub from your face using warm water, and follow with your favorite toner.

(7) Sugar and Salt Scrub

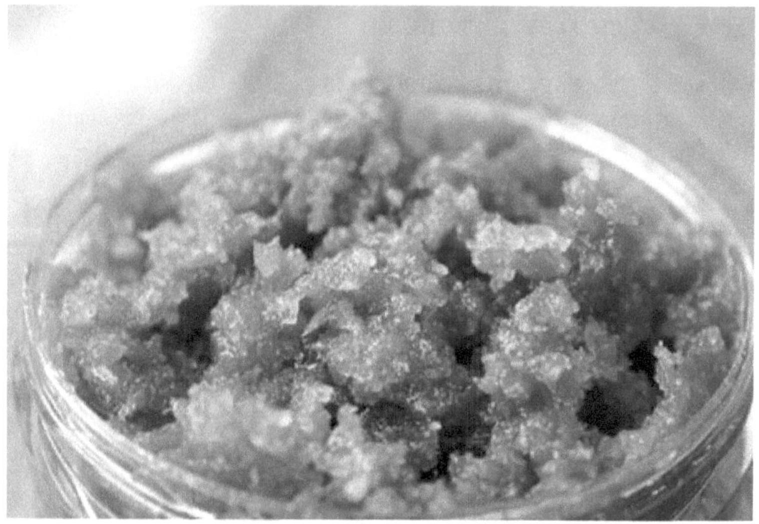

This scrub is ideal for dry, dull skin. A simple recipe using store-cupboard essentials that's great for the body (especially pre-holiday). Those with sensitive skin need to use with caution though, as it may be too abrasive.

Preparation Time: 5 mins

List of Ingredients:

- ½ cup brown sugar
- ¼ cup very fine salt
- 1 tablespoon extra-virgin olive oil

ooooooooooooooooooooooooooooooooooooo

Procedure:

1. First, prepare your skin by washing with warm water.

2. Combine all the ingredients in a small bowl and mix thoroughly.

3. Apply to the face, neck, and decolletage using wet fingertips in small, circular movements. Very gently, massage into the skin for 2-3 minutes.

4. Rinse off the excess scrub using warm water. Make sure your skin is free of any salt and sugar by using a damp cloth or cotton pad. Take care not to scratch your face. Pat dry with a clean, dry towel. Do not rub.

(8) Chamomile Scrub

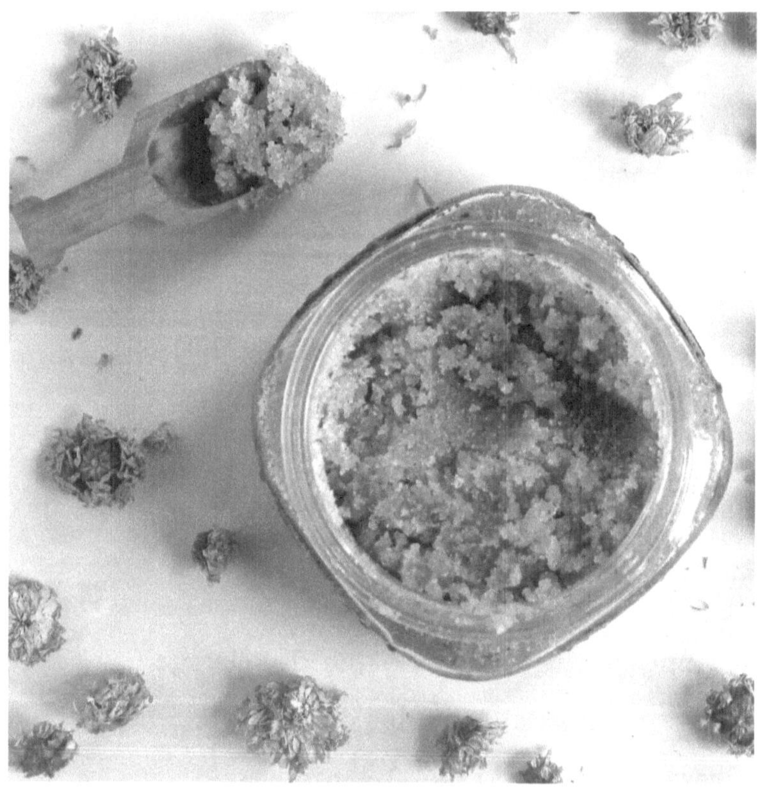

Going to a special event? This is the perfect scrub to give your skin a dewy glow for a special occasion. Why is it perfect? The sugar gently exfoliates, while chamomile soothes and calms, so your skin won't be pink or dry after use. This means you can apply your moisturizer and makeup immediately after, and benefit from the dewy glow straight away.

Preparation Time: 10 mins

List of Ingredients:

- 1 organic chamomile tea, tea bag
- ½ cup sugar
- ¼ cup olive oil

ooooooooooooooooooooooooooooooooooooo

Procedure:

1. Cut the top off of the tea bag and empty the contents into a small bowl. Add the remaining ingredients and stir well to combine.

2. Wet your clean skin with water and gently massage the scrub into your face. Rinse off with warm water and follow with cold water to re-close your pores.

3. Pat your skin dry with a soft towel and follow with your favorite moisturizer.

(9) Strawberry Lime Scrub

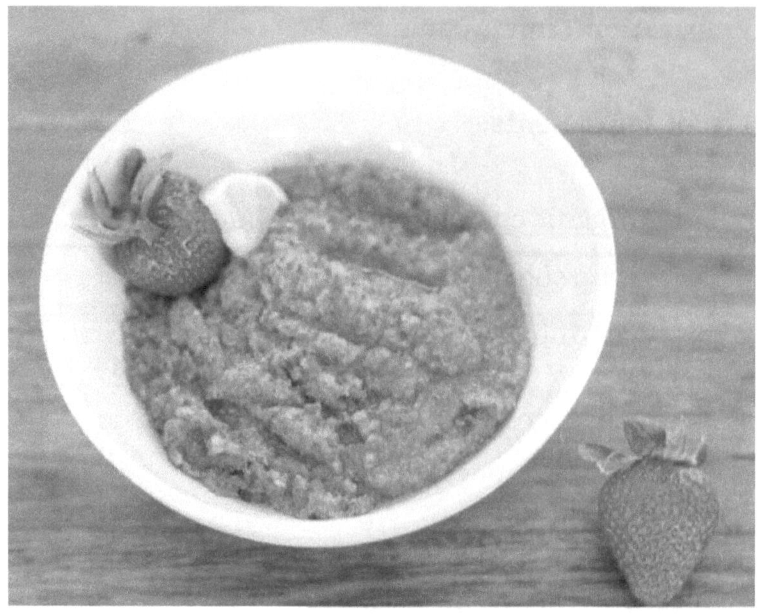

This fruity concoction is packed full of skin-brightening vitamins and minerals. Strawberries will improve skin tone, salt will gently exfoliate, while almond oil moisturizes. Not only will this scrub make your skin glow, but it also leaves behind a light, strawberry scent. Suitable for normal skin types only.

Preparation Time: 15 mins

List of Ingredients:

- 10 small, fresh strawberries
- ½ a lime, juiced
- 1 teaspoon almond oil
- 4 tablespoons sea salt

ooooooooooooooooooooooooooooooooooooooo

Procedure:

1. Pulse the strawberries in a food processor 5-6 times (do not puree them).

2. Transfer the strawberries to a bowl and add in the remaining ingredients. Stir well to combine.

3. Apply a tablespoon of scrub to clean, dry skin. Massage into your face using wet hands and small, circular motions. Allow the scrub to set on your skin for a few minutes before rinsing off.

4. Pat your skin dry with a soft towel.

5. Store any remaining scrub in a jar in the refrigerator*.

*Refrigerated scrub will keep for 7-10 days.

(10) Chocolate-Sugar Face Scrub

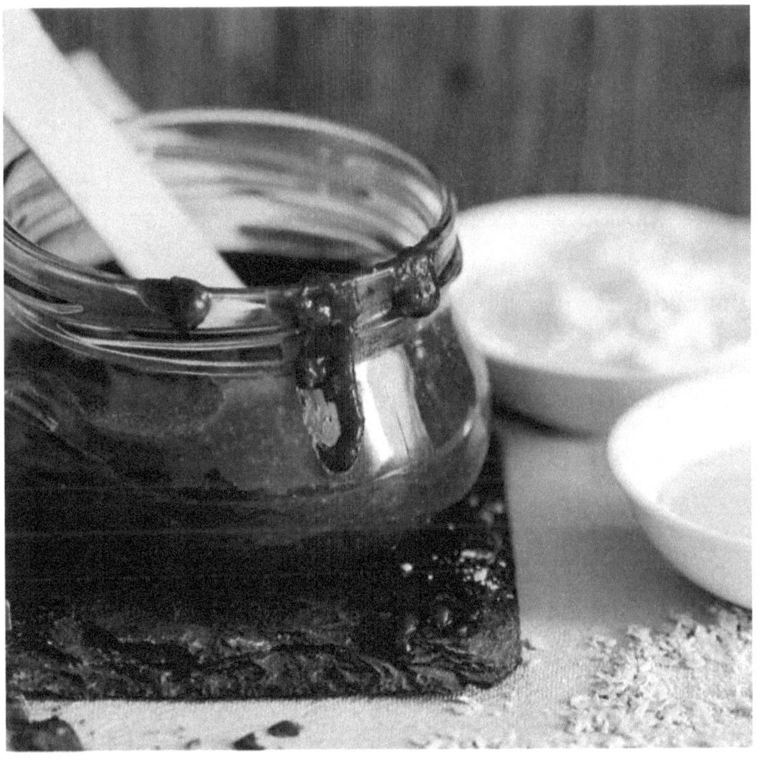

Cocoa powder is not simply for making hot drinks. Used as a facial scrub ingredient, it can ensure your complexion has a healthy glow. It is also great for removing a patchy tan. The good news is that it is suitable for all skin types.

Preparation Time: 14 mins

List of Ingredients:

- ¼ cup brown sugar
- ⅛ cup olive oil
- 1 tablespoon cocoa powder
- ¼ teaspoons vanilla extract

OOOOOOOOOOOOOOOOOOOOOOOOOOOOOOOOOOOOOO

Procedure:

1. First, thoroughly cleanse your skin using your cleanser of choice.

2. Combine all four ingredients in a small, clean bowl. Generously lather onto your clean face, rubbing in gentle, circular motions for no more than 60 seconds.

3. Allow the scrub to set on the skin for 10-12 minutes.

4. Rinse off with clean, warm water. Pat dry using a clean towel or cotton wool. Do not rub.

5. Allow the skin to rest for 2-3 hours before applying any makeup.

(11) Rosy Glow

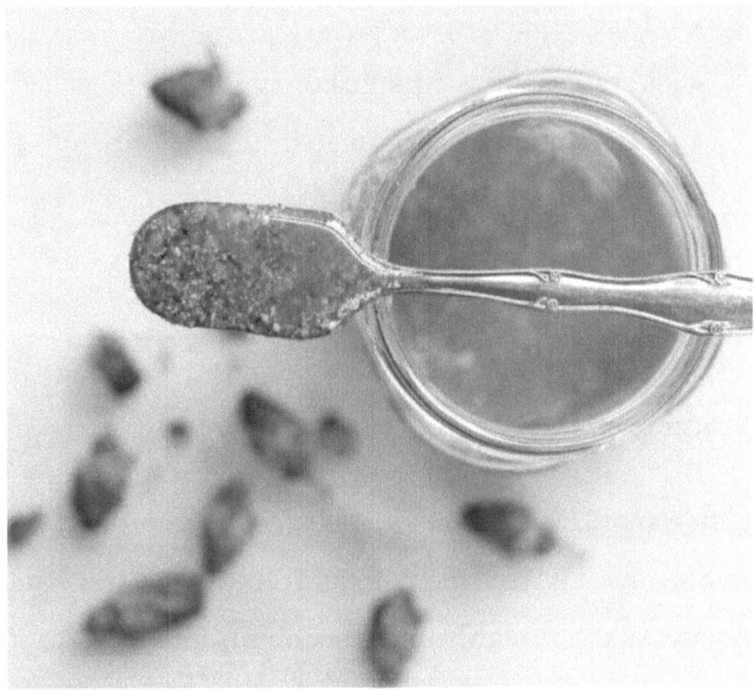

An aromatic facial scrub that will restore your skin to its healthy glow. Rosy not red. Rich in antioxidants, the rose water assists in cell turnover.

Preparation Time: 20 mins

List of Ingredients:

- 2 tablespoons coconut oil
- 1 tablespoon rose water
- ½ tablespoons organic honey
- 2½ tablespoons granulated sugar
- 1 small jar dried roses
- 1-2 drops rose essential oil

OOOOOOOOOOOOOOOOOOOOOOOOOOOOOOOOOOOOOOO

Procedure:

1. In a small, suitable bowl, melt the coconut oil in the microwave. When melted, add the rosewater and honey. Mix thoroughly until the mixture is a consistent color. Allow to cool.

2. Once cool, gradually add the granulated sugar while stirring with a small spoon. The mixture should be a soft paste with grains. Next, add the essential oil. Continue to stir.

3. Meanwhile, take a dried rose and add it to a glass of hot water. Allow the rose to steep for 2-3 seconds. When soft, scatter pieces on top of the scrub. These petals will help to add to the mixture's exfoliation properties.

4. Wash your face with warm water and pat dry. Using clean fingertips, gently massage the rose scrub into your skin using circular motions. Lightly work into the skin for 40 seconds.

5. Allow the scrub to set on the skin for 10-12 minutes.

6. Rinse off with clean, warm water. Pat dry using a clean towel or cotton wool. Do not rub.

(12) Coffee Face Scrub

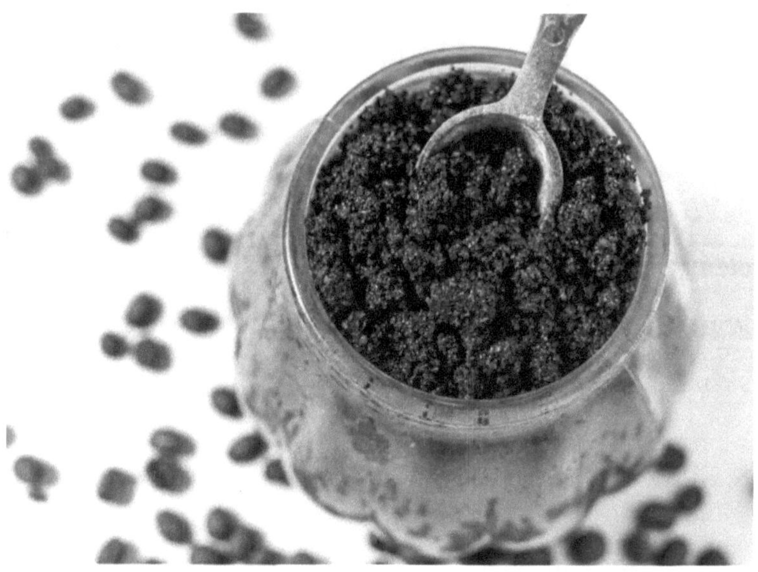

The coffee grounds will take care of all that dead skin. The coconut oil is great for moisturizing and the honey will help your skin retain that moisture. Your complexion will be so much brighter after using this scrub. This is an excellent recipe to use on the body too – just increase the volume of ingredients.

Preparation Time: 15 mins

List of Ingredients:

- 1½ teaspoons coffee grounds
- ⅓ teaspoons coconut oil
- 1 teaspoon organic honey

oooooooooooooooooooooooooooooooooooooo

Procedure:

1. First, thoroughly cleanse your skin using your cleanser of choice.

2. Combine all three ingredients in a small, clean bowl. Generously lather onto your clean face. Rub in gentle, circular motions for no more than 60 seconds.

3. Allow the scrub to set on the skin for 10-12 minutes.

4. Rinse off with clean, warm water. Pat dry using a clean towel or cotton wool. Do not rub.

5. Due to the small amount of coconut oil used in this scrub you will be able to apply makeup within 30 minutes or so.

(13) Nutmeg and Milk

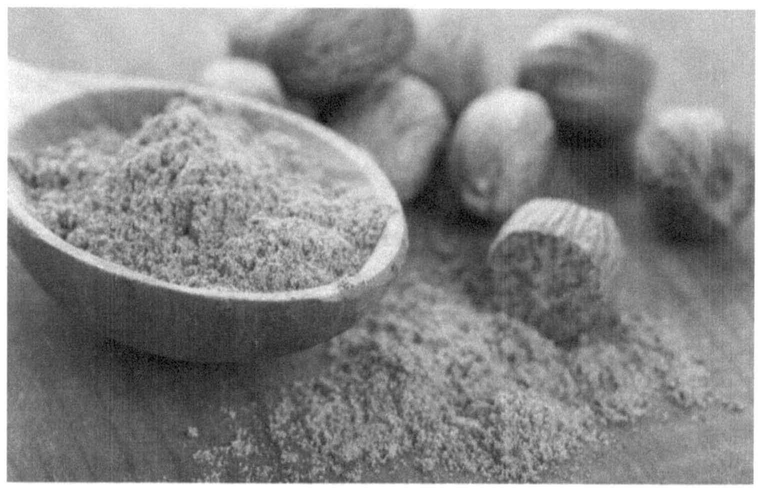

Combining milk and nutmeg in a scrub is a great way to put you on the road to a bright complexion. Not only will you clear away dead skin cells, but you'll also banish those blackheads. If possible, grind your own nutmeg rather than buying pre-ground nutmeg from the store.

Preparation Time: 4 mins

List of Ingredients:

- 2 tablespoons ground nutmeg
- 2 tablespoons full-fat milk

OOOOOOOOOOOOOOOOOOOOOOOOOOOOOOOOOOOOOOO

Procedure:

1. First, wash your face with warm water and pat dry.

2. In a small, clean bowl combine the nutmeg with milk. Using a spoon, mix until a paste forms.

3. Apply the scrub to the face in gentle, circular motions. Focus on any problem areas, especially around the chin, nose, and forehead. The nutmeg removes the dirt and impurities from the pores.

4. Rinse with warm water and pat dry using a clean towel. Do not rub.

(14) Creamy Brown Sugar Almond Scrub

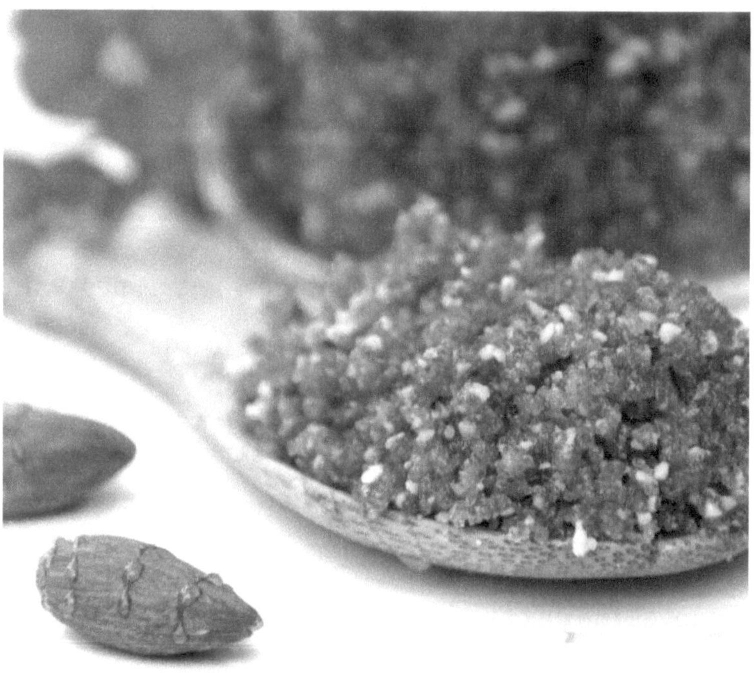

A buildup of dead skin cells is the most common reason behind dull skin. Massaging your face twice a week with this scrub will keep it looking bright and luminous, without drying it out.

Preparation Time: 15 mins

List of Ingredients:

- 1 cup almonds
- 3 tablespoons fresh cream
- 1 cup granulated sugar
- ½ cup light brown sugar
- 2 tablespoons olive oil

OOOOOOOOOOOOOOOOOOOOOOOOOOOOOOOOOOOOOOOO

Procedure:

1. Blitz the almonds in a food processor until totally ground.

2. Transfer the almonds to a bowl and add the remaining ingredients. Stir until well combined.

3. Massage a little of the scrub gently into your clean, dry skin for 1-2 minutes. Rinse off with warm water, and then splash your face with cold water to re-close your pores. Pat your face dry with a soft towel. Do not rub.

4. Store any remaining scrub in a sealable jar and keep in the refrigerator.

Chapter II - For Mature Skin

OOOOOOOOOOOOOOOOOOOOOOOOOOOOOOOOOOOOOOOOO

(15) Yogurt and Lime Juice Scrub

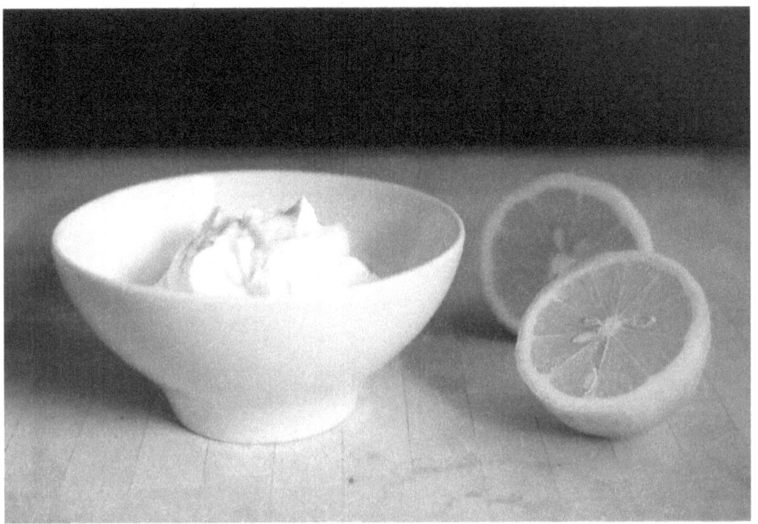

Citrus juices can help dry out acne, fight blackheads, and even prevent some skin breakouts. Lime juice combined with natural yogurt – the citric and lactic acids – refresh and renew. This inexpensive scrub, made from simple ingredients can moisturize, tone, fight wrinkles, and tighten the skin.

Preparation Time: 22 mins

List of Ingredients:

- 2 tablespoons natural, plain yogurt
- 1 tablespoon freshly-squeezed lime juice

OOOOOOOOOOOOOOOOOOOOOOOOOOOOOOOOOOOOOO

Procedure:

1. Prepare your skin by washing with warm water and patting dry.

2. In a small bowl, whip the yogurt and lime juice together to combine.

3. Using clean fingertips and working in circular movements, apply the mixture generously over your face and neck. Allow the scrub to dry on your face for no less than 15 minutes.

4. Once set, work from the outside of your face inwards and gently massage the scrub into your skin. This helps to stimulate the blood flow. Rinse with warm water and pat dry with a clean towel. Do not rub.

5. If you wish, you can apply a soothing lotion to help combat the acidity in the lime.

(16) Avocado, Grapefruit, and Sugar Scrub

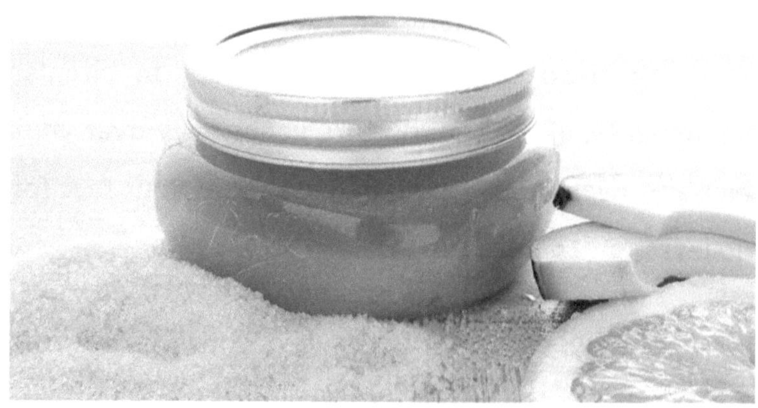

With special powers dedicated to battling nasty free radicals, grapefruit will have you looking 10 years younger in no time. Avocado oil prevents this mask from being too drying and won't block your pores.

Preparation Time: 15 mins

List of Ingredients:

- Juice of ½ fresh, yellow grapefruit
- 3 tablespoons avocado oil
- 1 cup granulated sugar

oooooooooooooooooooooooooooooooooooooo

Procedure:

1. Combine the grapefruit juice and oil in a small bowl and stir well to combine.

2. Add the sugar and stir a little (over-stirring will result in dissolved sugar and lessened the exfoliation).

3. Massage the scrub into your clean, dry skin, taking care to be extra-gentle around the eye area.

4. Rinse off with warm water and follow with a splash of cold water. Pat your face dry with a soft towel.

5. Store any remaining scrub in a jar in the refrigerator*.

*Refrigerated scrub will keep for 7-10 days.

(17) Tomato Sugar Face Scrub

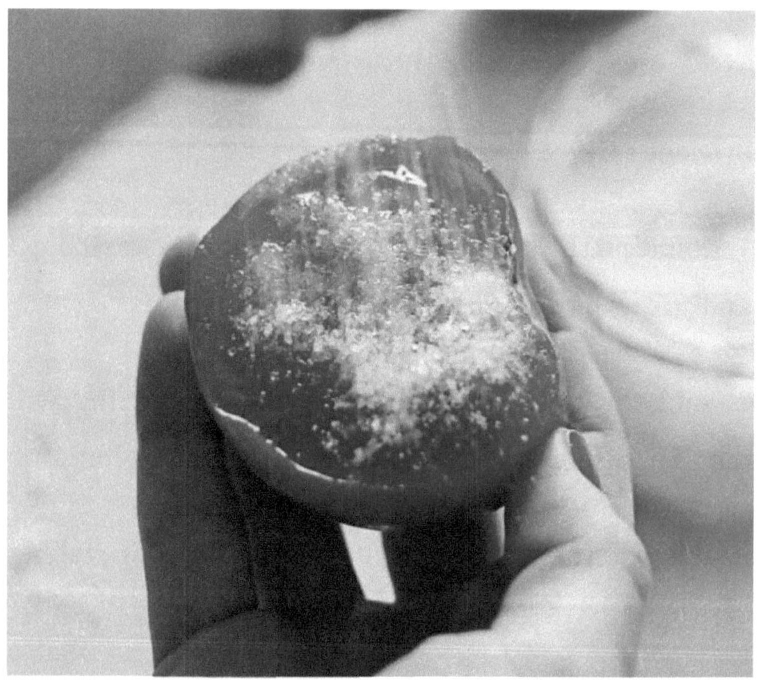

Tomatoes contain a naturally-occurring chemical called lycopene. It gives fruits and vegetables a red color and is an antioxidant that can help protect skin from harmful UV rays that damage skin's elasticity and cause wrinkles.

Preparation Time: 12 mins

List of Ingredients:

- 1 medium ripe tomato
- 1 tablespoon white sugar

OOOOOOOOOOOOOOOOOOOOOOOOOOOOOOOOOOOOOO

Procedure:

1. First, prepare your skin by washing with warm water and patting dry.

2. Add the sugar to a small plate. Slice the tomato crosswise and dip each slice in the white sugar, making sure it has adhered. Next, in circular motions, gently massage your face with the tomato halves. Avoid the eye area.

3. Allow your skin to rest for 8-10 minutes and then rinse with warm water. Pat dry using a clean towel. Do not rub.

(18) Blackberry and Walnut Scrub

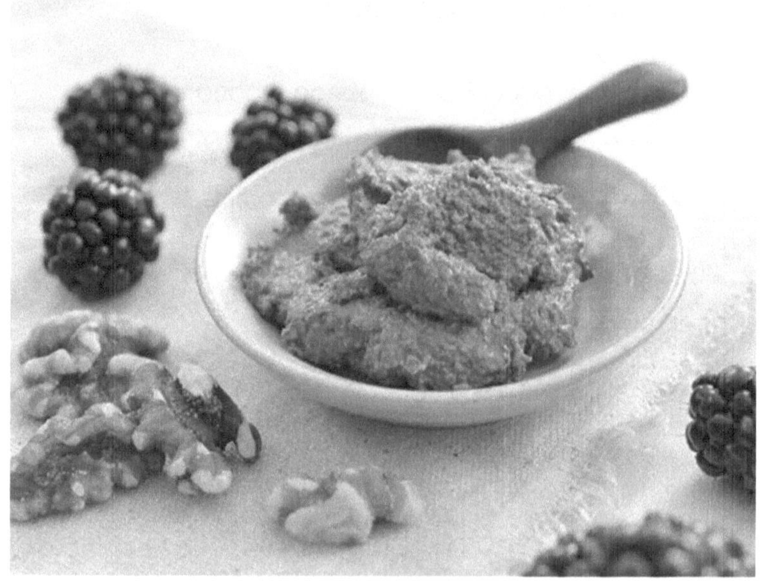

Two ingredients are all it takes to turn back the clock. For your face that is! Say goodbye to fine lines and wrinkles with this blackberry and walnut scrub. These powerful berries are bursting with antioxidants and vitamins which will reduce signs of aging and leave you with a youthful glow.

Preparation Time: 15 mins

List of Ingredients:

- ½ cup walnuts, roughly chopped
- ½ cup organic, fresh blackberries

OOOOOOOOOOOOOOOOOOOOOOOOOOOOOOOOOOOOOOO

Procedure:

1. Place the walnuts in a food processor and blitz until they are a fine powder. Set aside.

2. Add the blackberries to the empty processor and puree. Add the puree to the ground nuts and stir well to combine.

3. Moisten your skin with warm water. Massage the scrub gently into your skin for 2 minutes. Rinse away with warm water, pat your face dry with a soft towel, and follow with your preferred toner.

(19) Sugar Banana Scrub

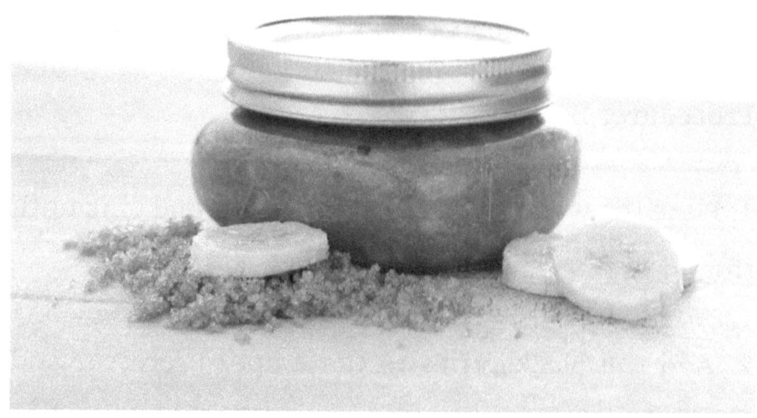

Bananas are literally Mother Nature's answer to Botox! Not only are they bursting with vitamins and nutrients, but they help to delay the aging process by protecting our skin from free radicals.

Preparation Time: 10 mins

List of Ingredients:

- 3 overripe bananas
- 1 cup light brown sugar

OOOOOOOOOOOOOOOOOOOOOOOOOOOOOOOOOOOOOOO

Procedure:

1. Mash the bananas in a bowl with a fork. Add the sugar and mix until combined.

2. Gently rub the mixture into your clean face. Allow the mask to sit for 10-15 minutes before rinsing your face well with warm water. Splash your face with cold water before patting dry with a soft towel. Wait 30-60 minutes before applying moisturizer or makeup.

3. Store any remaining scrub in a jar in the refrigerator*.

*Refrigerated scrub will keep for 7-10 days.

(20) Cherry Scrub

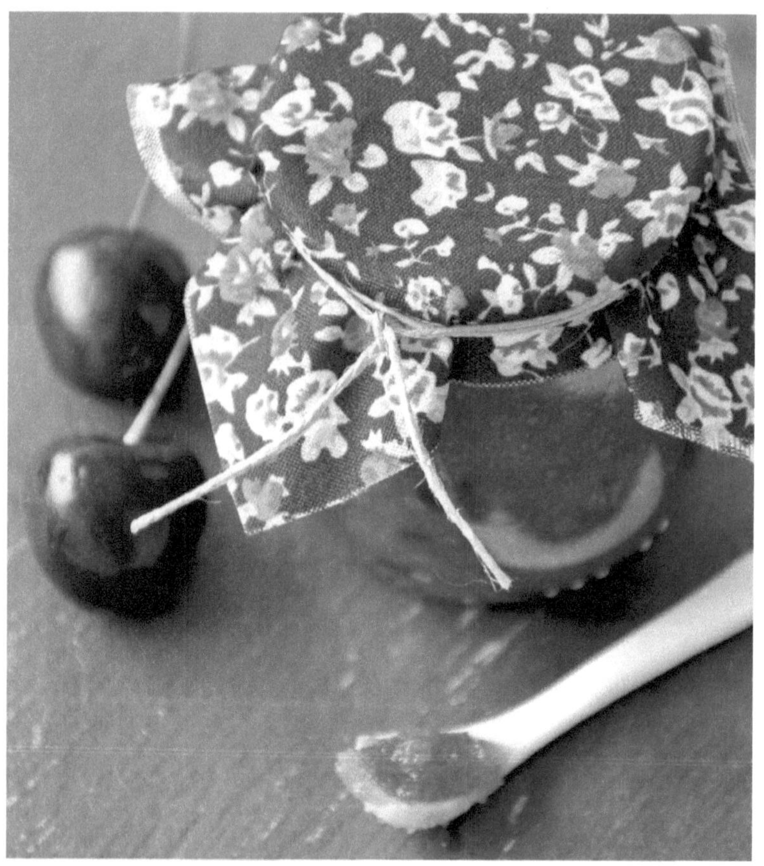

This scrub will rejuvenate dull, tired skin and give your complexion a pleasant glow. Cherries are rich in antioxidants to help reduce the signs of aging as they protect the skin from the damage caused by free radicals. It is also great as a face mask – simply omit the sugar.

Preparation Time: 28 mins

List of Ingredients:

- Handful of cherries, pitted
- 2 tablespoons of plain, natural yogurt
- 1 tablespoon granulated sugar

OOOOOOOOOOOOOOOOOOOOOOOOOOOOOOOOOOOOOOOOOO

Procedure:

1. First, prepare your skin by washing with warm water.

2. In a small bowl, using a fork to crush and pulp the cherries. Add the yogurt and sugar to the bowl and stir well to combine.

3. Apply the paste to your skin in gentle, circular movements for 2-3 minutes, massaging lightly. Allow the scrub to rest on the skin for 20 minutes.

4. Remove by washing in warm water. Pat dry with a clean towel. Do not rub.

(21) Strawberry and Honey Scrub

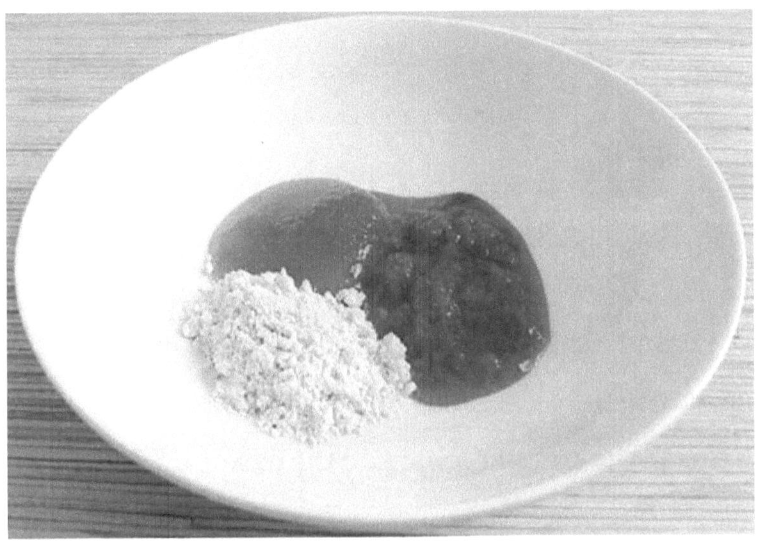

Who would have thought that strawberries could be so good for our skin? Did you know that they contain salicylic acid which is brilliant for anyone with an oily skin type? This scrub will help to achieve a healthy appearance, reduce wrinkles, and remove any excess oils.

Preparation Time: 20 mins

List of Ingredients:

- 3 ripe strawberries
- 2 teaspoons organic honey
- 2 tablespoons oatmeal

ooooooooooooooooooooooooooooooooooooo

Procedure:

1. First, wash your face with warm water and pat dry.

2. Grind the oatmeal in a coffee-grinder for approximately 5 seconds. In a medium bowl, use a fork to mash the strawberries. Add the oatmeal to the bowl.

3. Next, stir in the honey until completely blended.

4. Gently massage the scrub into the face, using circular motions for 5-6 minutes. Allow the scrub to rest for 8-10 minutes. Wash face using warm water and pat dry with clean towel.

(22) Egg Scrub

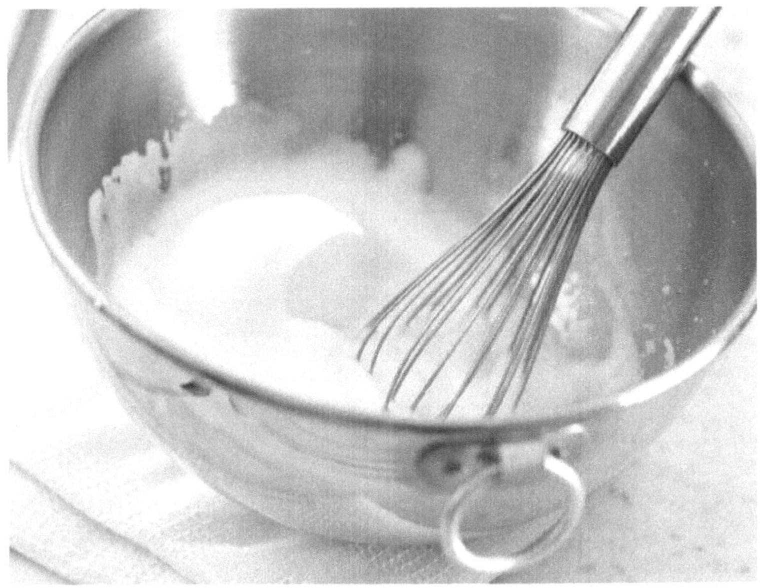

Egg, really? Yes! Packed full of protein, eggs have toning and tightening properties. They're also packed with B2 which helps to protect your face from other environmental stressors.

Preparation Time: 15 mins

List of Ingredients:

- 1 large egg
- 1 teaspoon freshly squeezed lemon juice.
- ½ teaspoons cane sugar

oooooooooooooooooooooooooooooooooooooo

Procedure:

1. Crack the egg into a small bowl and beat well. Add the lemon juice and sugar and stir well.

2. Use a clean makeup brush to apply the mixture to your face evenly.

3. Wait for the scrub to dry. Wet your hands a little and gently massage the dried scrub into your skin for 2-3 minutes.

4. Rinse off with warm water. Your face may be a little red after rinsing, which is normal. Allow your skin to calm a little before applying moisturizer or makeup.

(23) Spiced Mocha Scrub*

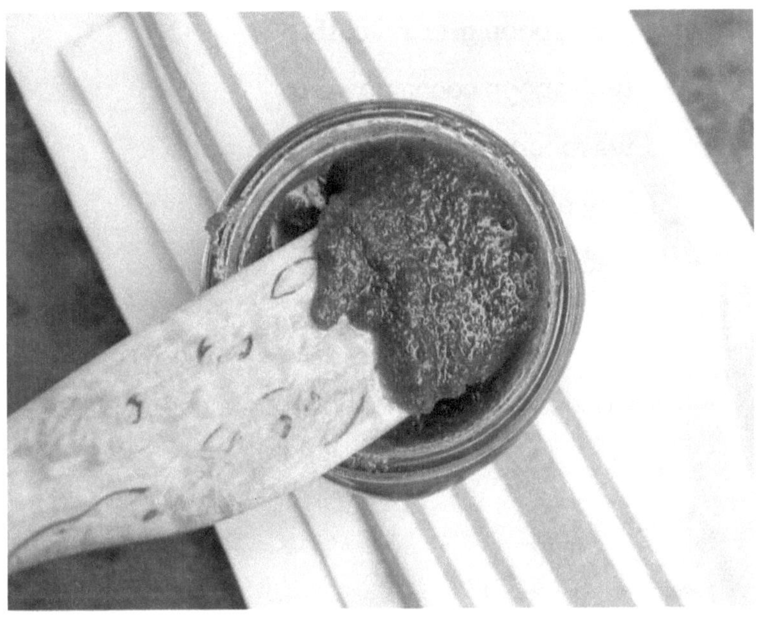

Surprisingly enough, spices can be helpful to our complexion. There are antioxidants in cinnamon that can help to smooth skin that is rough, and assist in the prevention of acne. Ginger has antiseptic properties and helps to cleanse and fight aging. While nutmeg can help to restore moisture.

Preparation Time: 4 mins

List of Ingredients:

- 1 cup sugar
- 1 tablespoon ground coffee
- 1 tablespoon cocoa powder
- 1 teaspoon cinnamon
- Large pinch nutmeg
- Large pinch ginger
- ¼-½ cup jojoba oil or almond oil

OOOOOOOOOOOOOOOOOOOOOOOOOOOOOOOOOOOOOOO

Procedure:

1. First, wash face with warm water and pat dry.

2. In a medium, clean bowl combine the sugar, coffee, cocoa powder, and the three spices. Gradually add the jojoba oil (you can substitute almond oil here) and whisk until totally combined.

3. Using clean fingertips, apply a generous amount to the face in circular movements, avoiding the eye area. Lightly massage into the skin for 60 seconds. You should never leave cinnamon on the skin for too long as it can act as an irritant.

4. Rinse off with warm water and pat dry using a clean towel.

*This scrub is not suitable for those with nut allergies. A patch test is recommended.

(24) Honey and Lemon Scrub

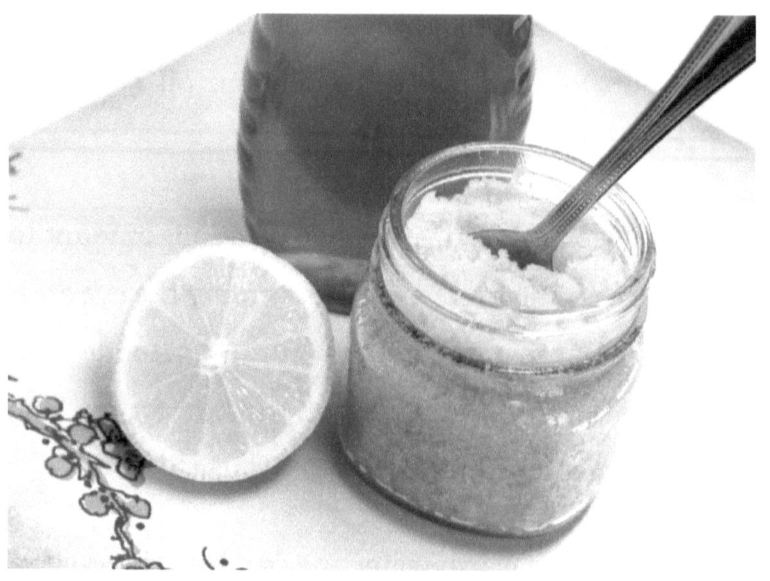

Coconut has great antioxidant properties which can help to keep your complexion looking youthful. Honey assists with moisture absorption, lemon brightens, and sea salt exfoliates; a great natural pick-me-up for dry skin.

Preparation Time: 30 mins

List of Ingredients:

- 1 teaspoon organic coconut oil
- 1 teaspoon organic honey
- 1½ teaspoons sea salt
- ⅓ teaspoons freshly-squeezed lemon juice

OOOOOOOOOOOOOOOOOOOOOOOOOOOOOOOOOOOOOOO

Procedure:

1. In a small, clean bowl combine the coconut oil and honey. Gradually, add the lemon juice, a drop at a time. The scrub should be soft but not liquid. Finally, add the sea salt and stir gently to combine, ensuring an even consistency. Place the bowl in the refrigerator to solidify.

2. Once the scrub is solid, thoroughly rinse your skin and pat dry.

3. Scrub the paste lightly onto your clean face. Rub gently in circular motions for no more than 30 seconds. Due to the acidity in the lemon juice avoid the eye area.

4. Rinse off with clean, warm water taking care to totally remove the coconut oil, which may feel a little tacky. Remember though, the fine layer of oil helps to make your skin glow. Pat dry using a clean towel or cotton wool. Do not rub.

(25) Spiced-Apple Chia Scrub

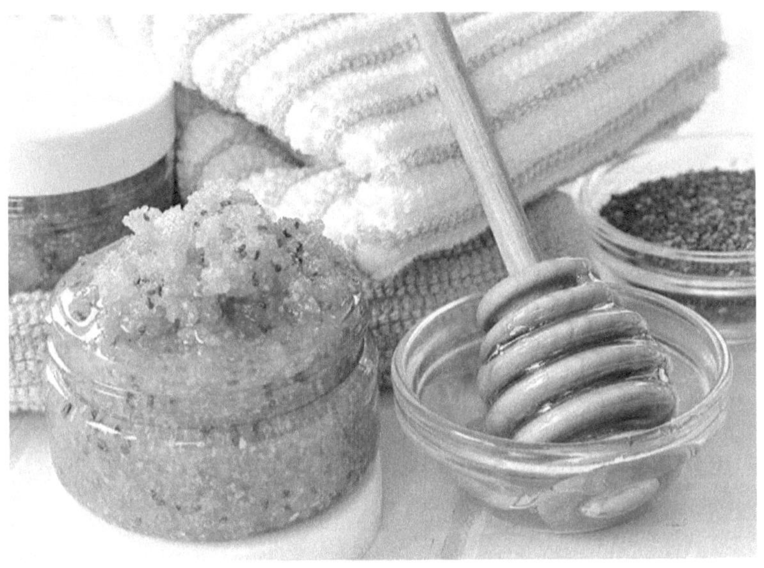

There's no need to break the bank in the quest for more youthful-looking skin. This scrub uses cheap ingredients produced by Mother Nature, not a laboratory. Alpha hydroxy acid, polyphenols, and flavonoids are all totally natural chemicals that will soothe, brighten, and plump up tired skin for a younger-looking complexion.

Preparation Time: 20 mins

List of Ingredients:

- ½ cup organic green apple, chopped
- 2 tablespoons chia seeds
- 2 tablespoons runny, organic honey

OOOOOOOOOOOOOOOOOOOOOOOOOOOOOOOOOOOOOOO

Procedure:

1. Add all ingredients into a food processor and blitz until you have a smooth puree. Add a drop of water if the mixture needs loosening. Transfer to a small bowl.

2. Allow the scrub to sit for 5-10 minutes in the refrigerator.

3. Apply the scrub to clean, dry skin and slowly massage into your face for 1-2 minutes. Rinse away with warm water, pat your face dry with a soft towel, and follow with your preferred toner.

(26) Raw Manuka Mask with Frankincense

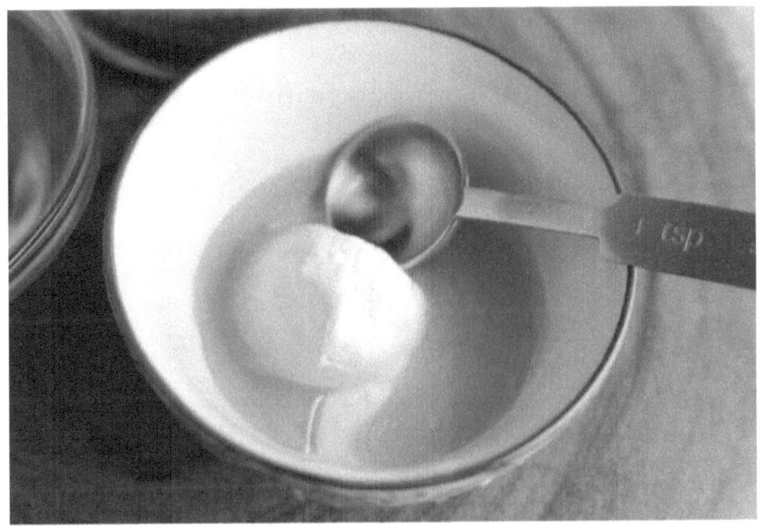

This mask is packed with anti-aging essential oils, the most notable being frankincense. Frankincense oil is proven to reduce the unwanted appearance of age and sun spots, not to mention wrinkles. Focus this mask on the areas where you want to increase elasticity, around the jowls for example.

Preparation Time: 10 mins

List of Ingredients:

- ½ tablespoons manuka honey
- 1 tablespoon baking soda
- 1 drop frankincense oil
- 1 drop lavender oil
- Rosewater (for after cleansing)*

OOOOOOOOOOOOOOOOOOOOOOOOOOOOOOOOOOOOOOOO

Procedure:

1. In a small bowl, add the baking soda and manuka honey. Stir well until it forms a paste. Drop in the essential oils and stir well to combine.

2. Wash your face with warm water to open the pores.

3. Gently massage the scrub into your skin for 4-6 minutes using circular motions.

4. Rinse your skin with warm water and splash with rosewater.

*This mask is alkaline; splashing your face with rosewater after rinsing will naturally restore your skin's pH balance.

Chapter III - For Problem Skin

OOOOOOOOOOOOOOOOOOOOOOOOOOOOOOOOOOOOOOOOOO

(27) Zucchini Scrub

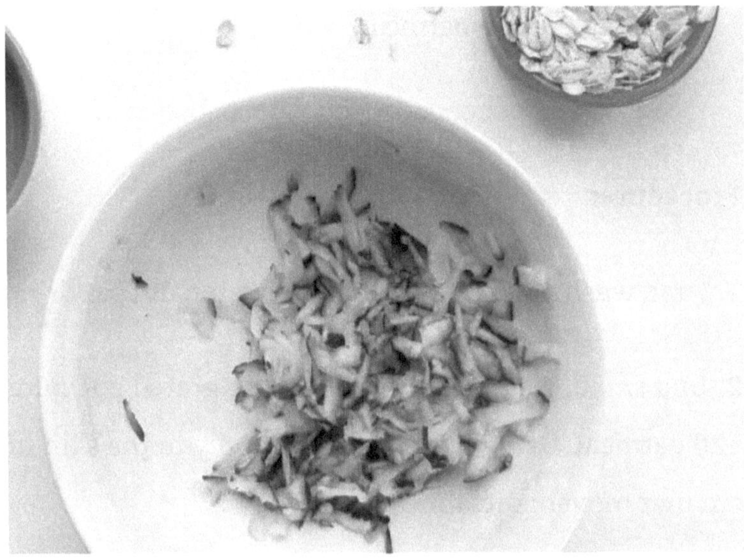

This is a cooling and refreshing scrub for skin that is in need of purification. Suitable for all skin types but particularly good for problematic complexions. This scrub can also be adapted to a face mask; simply steam the zucchini, rather than using it raw.

Preparation Time: 25 mins

List of Ingredients:

- 2 tablespoons zucchini, grated
- 1 tablespoon oatmeal

ooooooooooooooooooooooooooooooooooooooo

Procedure:

1. First, wash your face with warm water and pat dry.

2. In a small, clean bowl combine the grated zucchini and oatmeal. Using wet fingertips, apply to the skin in circular movements for 2-3 minutes.

3. Allow to rest on the skin for 15-20 minutes. Rinse off with warm water and pat dry with a clean towel.

(28) Apple and Sage Scrub

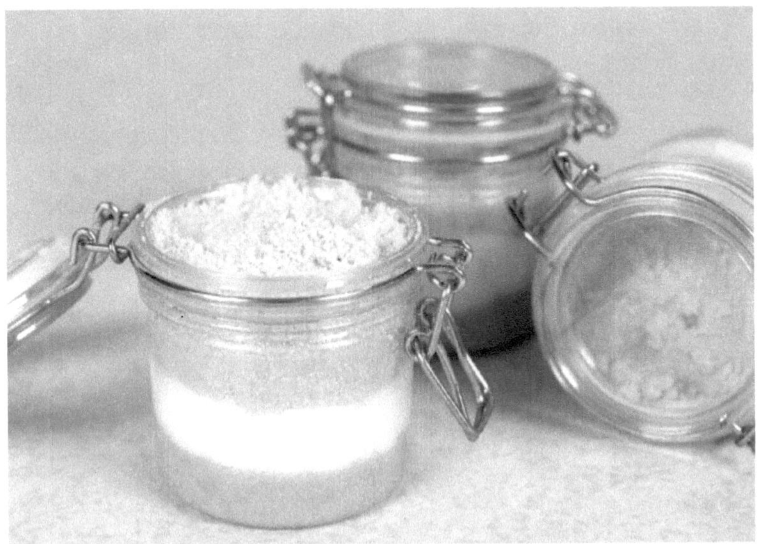

Oily skin sufferers will love this citrus-scented scrub. The fruit acids in apple and lemon exfoliate and remove oil, while sage closes and tightens pores, thanks to its natural astringent properties.

Preparation Time: 20 mins

List of Ingredients:

- 1 tablespoon organic applesauce
- 1 teaspoon freshly-squeezed lemon juice
- 1 teaspoon dried sage

OOOOOOOOOOOOOOOOOOOOOOOOOOOOOOOOOOOOOOO

Procedure:

1. Combine all ingredients in a small bowl and stir well to combine.

2. Gently massage the scrub into your clean, dry skin for 2-3 minutes. Rinse off with warm water, followed by cold. Pat your face dry with a soft towel*.

*Your skin may feel a little tight after rinsing, that is normal. After 10 minutes, follow with your preferred moisturizer.

(29) Witch Hazel and Clay Deep-Cleansing Scrub

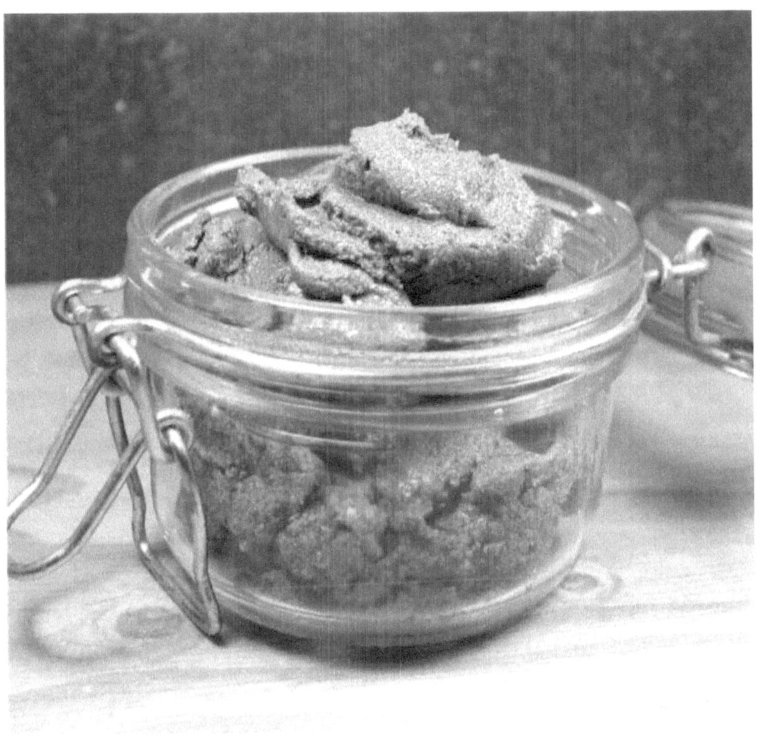

Witch hazel is a natural ingredient which acts as a gentle astringent to tighten pores, while clay sinks deep into the skin to pull out dirt and impurities as it is rinsed away. This scrub is ideal for anyone suffering from oily skin and, consequentially, pimples or blackheads. Use once a week after showering for best results.

Preparation Time: 20 mins

List of Ingredients:

- 1 tablespoon witch hazel
- 1 teaspoon bentonite clay
- 2 drops lemon oil
- 1 teaspoon light brown sugar

OOOOOOOOOOOOOOOOOOOOOOOOOOOOOOOOOOOOOOO

Procedure:

1. In a small, plastic bowl, combine all ingredients and stir well to combine with a wooden spoon.

2. Wash your face well with warm - just hot water* to open pores and pat dry with a towel,

3. Apply the scrub to your face and allow to sit for 15 minutes.

4. Wet your hands with cold water and massage the dried scrub into your skin for 2-3 minutes. Wash away with warm water, followed by cold. Pat your face dry with a soft towel,

*While warm water will open pores, it is best to use this scrub after a hot shower when your pores are at their most open. This will allow the clay to sink deeper for improved impurity removal.

(30) Avocado and Brown Sugar Scrub

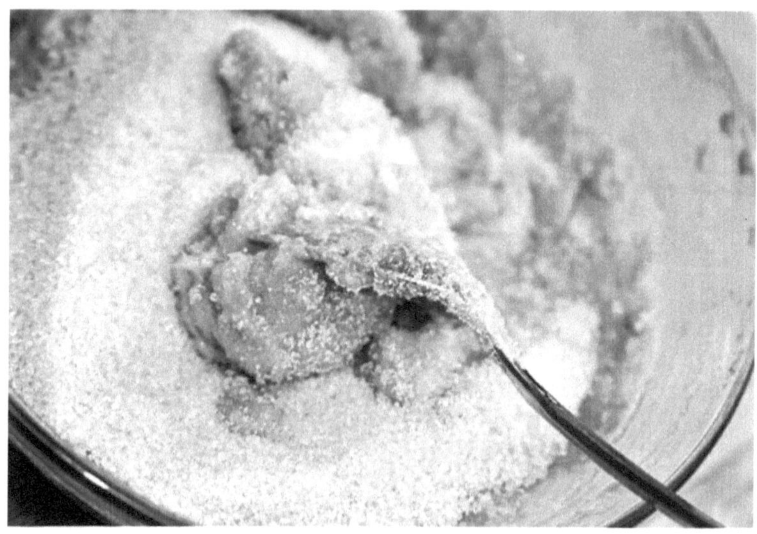

Finally, a scrub suitable for sensitive skin! Avocado is rich in Vitamin E and, whether we digest it or apply it externally to our skin, the benefits remain the same.

Preparation Time: 9 mins

List of Ingredients:

- ½ cup brown sugar
- ¼ cup avocado oil
- I small cucumber

OOOOOOOOOOOOOOOOOOOOOOOOOOOOOOOOOOOOOOO

Procedure:

1. First, wash your makeup-free face with warm water and pat dry.

2. In a small, clean, glass bowl mix the brown sugar with the avocado oil. In a blender, blitz the cucumber. Add the sugar-oil mixture to the cucumber mixture. Transfer to a bowl and stir until combined.

3. Using clean fingertips and circular movements, gently massage the scrub into your face and neck. (Don't be afraid to apply to your lips as well. They deserve a treat too!)

4. Allow the scrub to sit for 2-3 minutes. Wash off with warm water and pat dry with a clean towel. Do not rub.

(31) Sensitive Almond Clay Scrub

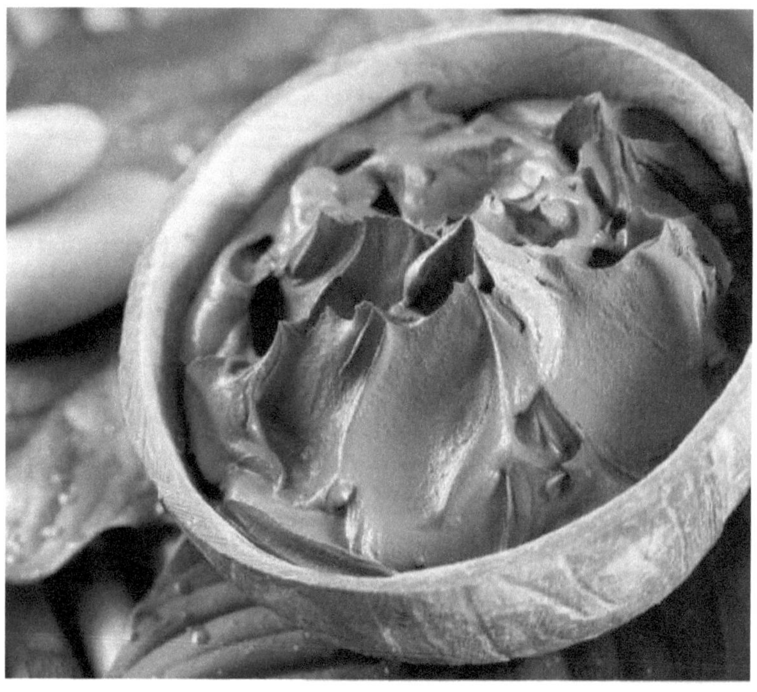

This scrub is free from abrasive sugar or salt, making it perfect for hypersensitive skin. It makes use of only powders, including bentonite clay which will deeply cleanse your skin without irritating it. Not only that, but because it is solely powder (you add water when you want to use it) you can make this scrub ahead and use it for months!

Preparation Time: 20 mins

List of Ingredients:

- ½ cup finely ground almond meal
- ½ cup bentonite clay
- 2 tablespoons organic powdered whole-milk

OOOOOOOOOOOOOOOOOOOOOOOOOOOOOOOOOOOOOOOO

Procedure:

1. Combine all ingredients in a large mason jar. Screw on the lid and shake well until all powders are combined.

2. When you are ready to use, take a tablespoon of powder in the palm of your hand. Add a few drops of lukewarm water, to make a paste. Massage the paste into your skin for 1-2 minutes. Allow the paste to sit and dry for 5-10 minutes. Rinse off with warm water, followed by cold.

3. Allow skin to calm for 5-10 minutes before applying your preferred moisturizer.

(32) Blackhead Removal Scrub

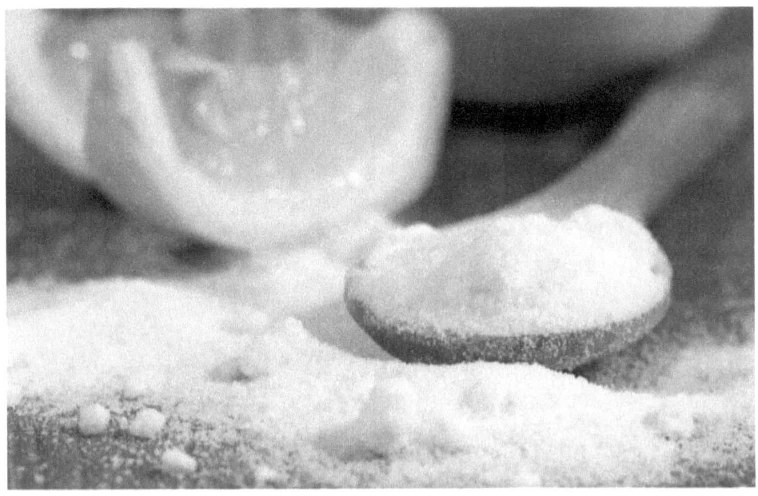

Who doesn't hate pesky blackheads? Now there's a simple solution that doesn't involve expensive creams or painful, sticky pore strips. This blackhead removal scrub contains only two ingredients and can be whipped up in under 2 minutes! For best results, apply this scrub after a hot shower when your pores are open.

Preparation Time: 30 mins

List of Ingredients:

- 2 tablespoons baking soda
- 6 teaspoons freshly-squeezed orange juice
- Witch hazel (to tone)

OOOOOOOOOOOOOOOOOOOOOOOOOOOOOOOOOOOOOOOO

Procedure:

1. Combine both ingredients in a small bowl and mix well.

2. Start by washing your face with plenty of warm to medium-hot water*. Pat your face dry and apply the scrub to your face, focusing on your T-zone.

3. Allow the mask to harden for approximately 15-20 minutes.

4. Wet your hands with cold water and rub the dried mask into your face using small, circular motions.

5. Rinse your face thoroughly with cold water and follow with a witch hazel toner.

* For best results, use this scrub after a hot shower when your pores are most open; this allows the scrub to get deep down to best remove blackheads.

(33) Peach Scrub

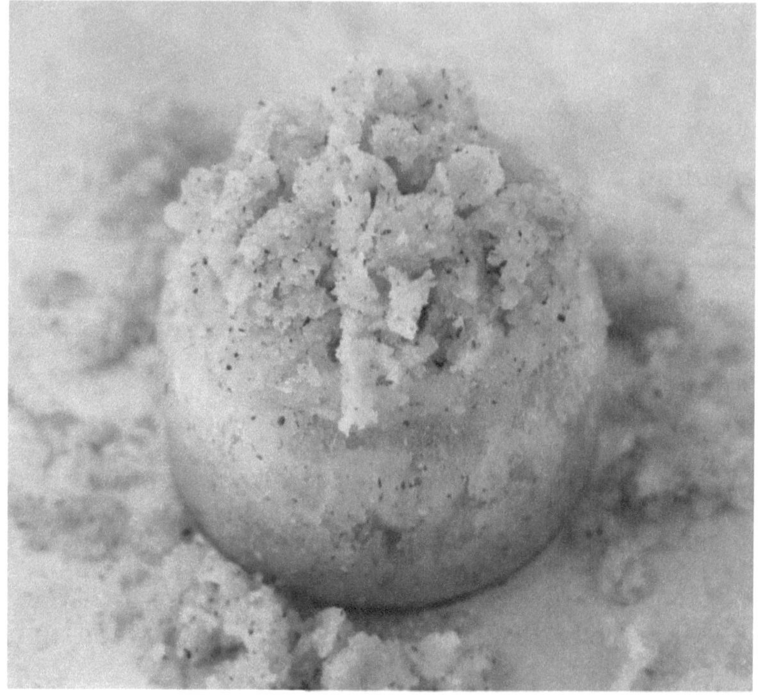

Scrub your way to brighter, pimple-free skin. The alpha hydroxy acid in this sweet fruit promotes new cell growth while removing old, dead cells. This is great news for acne-scarred skin! Not only that, after using 1-2 times a week for a month you'll notice a smoother, clearer, brighter, and blackhead-free complexion, thanks to the scrubs high levels of vitamin A and C.

Preparation Time: 15 mins

List of Ingredients:

- 1 over-ripe, fresh peach
- ½ tablespoons coconut oil
- ½ tablespoons runny honey
- 1 tablespoon light brown sugar

OOOOOOOOOOOOOOOOOOOOOOOOOOOOOOOOOOOOOOOO

Procedure:

1. Add the peaches to a food processor and blitz until pureed. Transfer the peach puree to a small bowl and add the remaining ingredients. Stir to combine.

2. Apply to clean, dry skin using a gentle, massaging action for 2-3 minutes. Allow the scrub to sit for a few minutes before washing off with warm water, followed by cold.

3. Pat face dry with a soft towel and apply your preferred moisturizer after 5-10 minutes.

4. Store any leftover scrub in a jar in the refrigerator*.

*Peach scrub will last for one week in the refrigerator.

(34) Blueberry and Honey

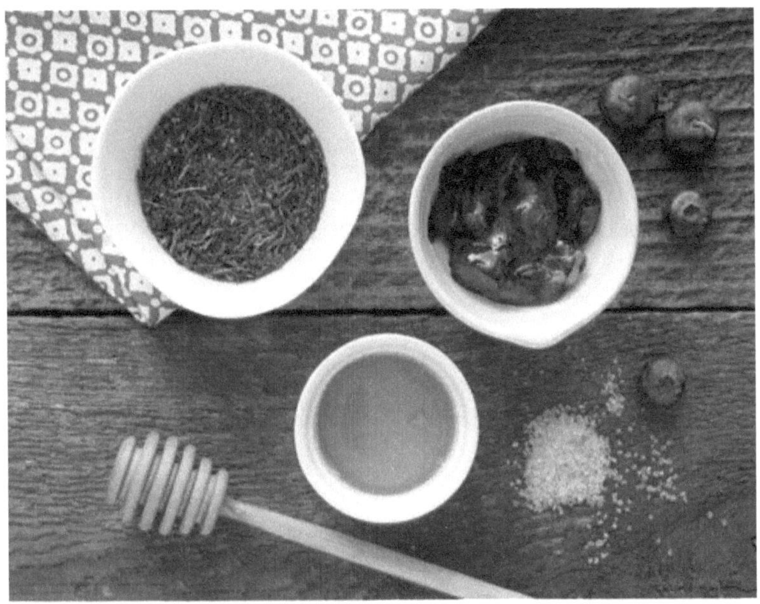

Literally bursting with antioxidants and Vitamin C, blueberries are sent from nature to work their magic on blemishes and boils. The same also goes for honey which has amazing anti-inflammatory properties. Matcha can have positive long-term effects on our skin's elasticity and luminosity.

Preparation Time: 25 mins

List of Ingredients:

- ⅓ cup fresh blueberries
- 2 tablespoons honey
- ½ teaspoons Matcha tea
- 1 teaspoon super-fine sugar

OOOOOOOOOOOOOOOOOOOOOOOOOOOOOOOOOOOOOO

Procedure:

1. First, wash your face in warm water and pat dry with a clean towel.

2. Thoroughly wash the blueberries in cold water, before putting them in a small bowl. Using a fork, mash them to a pulp. Next, add the honey, Matcha tea, and white sugar. Stir well to combine.

3. With clean fingertips, gently apply a generous layer to the face, neck, and decolletage area. Massage gently into the skin using circular movements. Allow the scrub to sit for 12-15 minutes.

4. Rinse well with warm water and pat dry with a clean towel. Do not rub.

(35) Oats-So-Simple Scrub

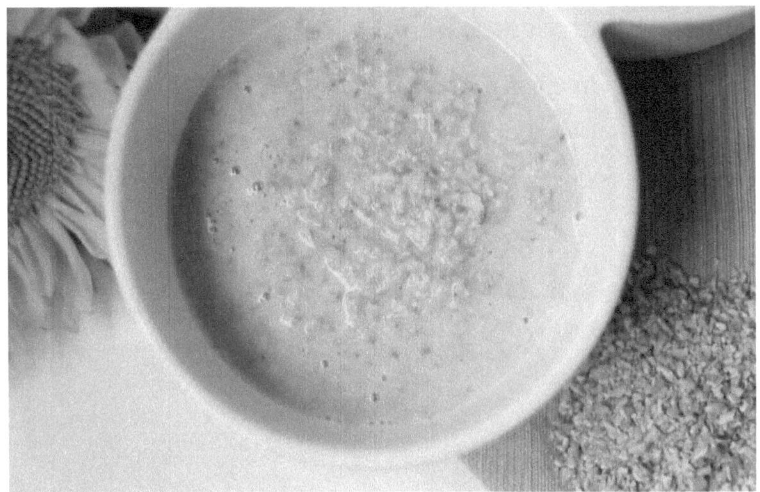

Skin can become dry for a lot of different reasons. Wind, sun, and even air-conditioning can cause our skin to break out in dry patches, making it feel tight and uncomfortable. A simple scrub containing olive oil can really help to restore balance.

Preparation Time: 15 mins

List of Ingredients:

- ¼ cup uncooked oats
- ⅛ cup organic honey
- ⅛ cup virgin olive oil

OOOOOOOOOOOOOOOOOOOOOOOOOOOOOOOOOOOOOO

Procedure:

1. In a food processor/blender on a medium setting, pulse the uncooked oats. (The oats will act as the exfoliating agent so they need to be broken, rather than powdered.) Transfer the oats to a small - medium, clean, glass bowl.

2. Using a spoon, stir in the organic honey and olive oil, a little at a time.

3. Wash your face using a cleanser of choice. With clean, wet fingertips, smear a layer of scrub onto the skin and, in circular motions, lightly massage into the face for 60 seconds or so.

4. For additional moisture, leave on the skin for 7-10 minutes. Rinse with cold water and pat the skin dry with a clean towel. Do not rub.

(36) Clarifying Honey/Lemon Scrub

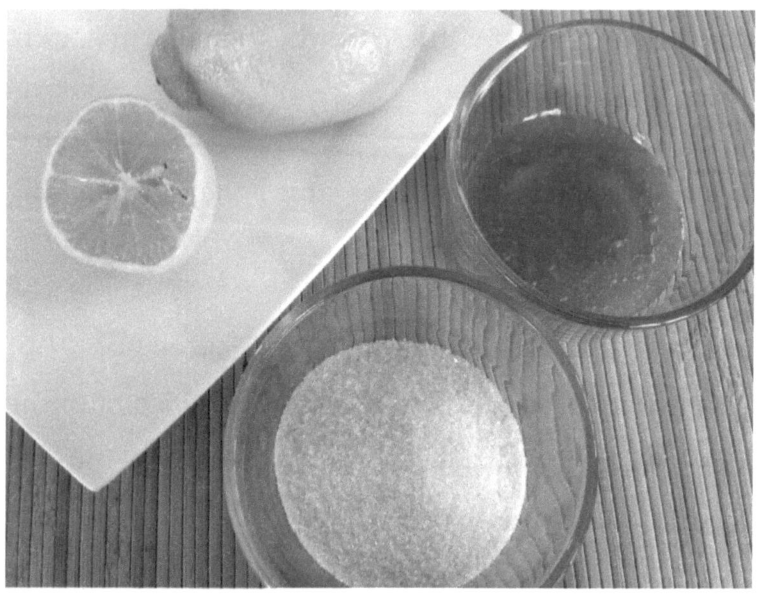

Honey is known for its powerful antimicrobial and antioxidant properties. Combined with clarifying lemon and natural exfoliant, cane sugar, this is the perfect scrub for pimple-prone skin. You'll be on the road to a clear complexion in no time.

Preparation Time: 10 mins

List of Ingredients:

- ½ teaspoons organic honey
- 1 ¼ teaspoons cane sugar
- Some freshly-squeezed lemon juice

OOOOOOOOOOOOOOOOOOOOOOOOOOOOOOOOOOOOOO

Procedure:

1. Combine all ingredients in a small bowl and mix well with a spoon.

2. Wet your clean skin with warm water to make the scrub easier to massage into your skin.

3. Gently rub the mixture into your skin using small, circular motions. Rinse it off with warm water, then follow with cold water*. Pat your face dry. Do not rub.

*Depending on the brand of honey you use, your scrub may be a little sticky. Take care to thoroughly rinse your face to remove all traces of the scrub. Your skin may be a little pink after exfoliating, that's normal. Wait for your skin to calm before applying any further products.

(37) Maple Scrub

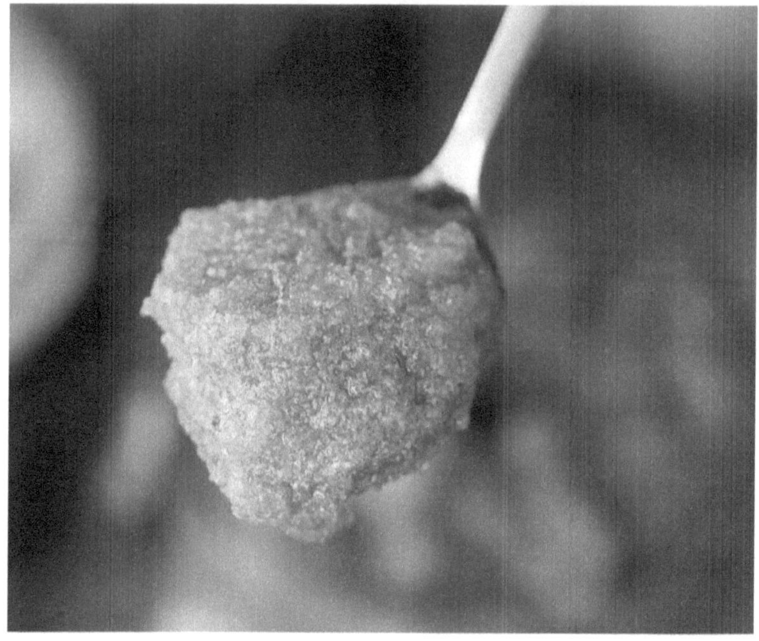

High in antioxidants and zinc, maple syrup is impressively hydrating. Turmeric has antibacterial properties and can help combat acne and excessive oiliness. Olive oil will hydrate and soften the skin.

Preparation Time: 5 mins

List of Ingredients:

- 4 tablespoons ground oats
- 4 tablespoons pure maple syrup
- Big pinch of turmeric
- 1 tablespoon virgin olive oil

oooooooooooooooooooooooooooooooooooooooo

Procedure:

1. First, wash your face with warm water and pat dry.

2. In a small, clean bowl combine all four ingredients and mix into a thick paste.

3. Using damp, clean fingertips, gently apply the scrub using small, circular movements for 2-3 minutes.

4. Rinse off with a damp cloth or cotton pad and pat dry with a clean towel. Do not rub.

(38) Gentle Oat and Green Tea Scrub

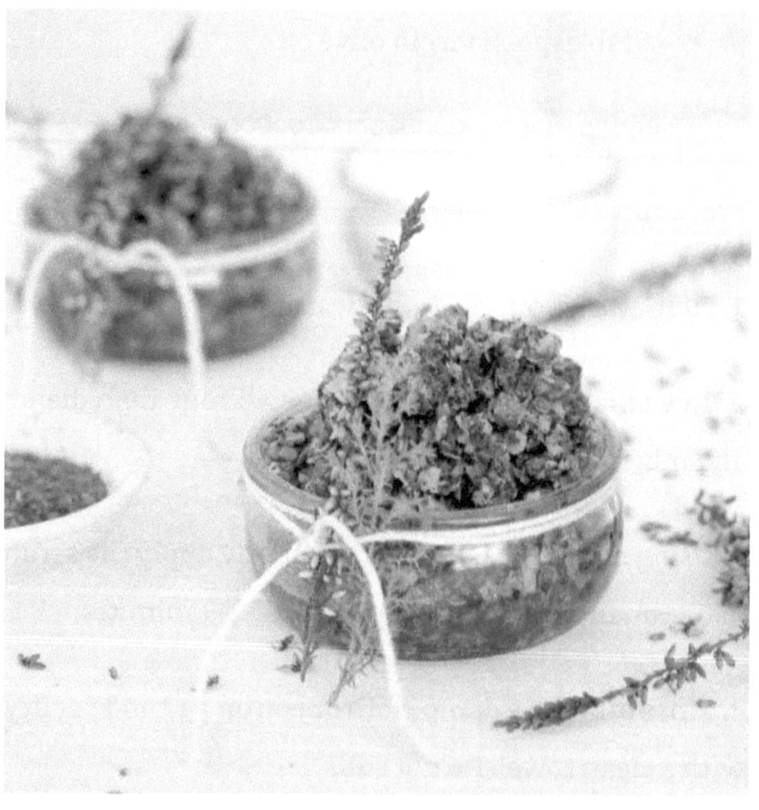

Many people with sensitive skin feel they should avoid scrubs at all cost. Although it is correct to stay away from overly abrasive products, it is still important to deeply cleanse your skin to remove impurities. This super-gentle oat and green tea mask will clean your skin and assist with skin conditions such as eczema; its anti-inflammatory properties mean it will do so without irritating your complexion.

Preparation Time: 20 mins

List of Ingredients:

- 5 organic green tea teabags
- ¾ cups rolled oats
- ½ cup sugar
- 2 tablespoons organic honey
- ¾ cup olive oil
- 15 drops vanilla essence
- 5 drops lavender oil

OOOOOOOOOOOOOOOOOOOOOOOOOOOOOOOOOOOOOO

Procedure:

1. Combine all of the ingredients in a medium bowl and stir well to combined.

2. Wet your clean face and neck with warm water. Massage the scrub gently into your face, neck, and even your chest (optional).

3. Allow to sit for 8-10 minutes before washing off with warm water, followed by cold. Allow your skin to settle for 30 minutes before applying a gentle moisturizing cream.

4. Store any remaining scrub in a jar in the refrigerator*.

* Scrub will last for up to 21 days in a refrigerator, but is best applied when fresh.

(39) Lavender and Vanilla Scrub

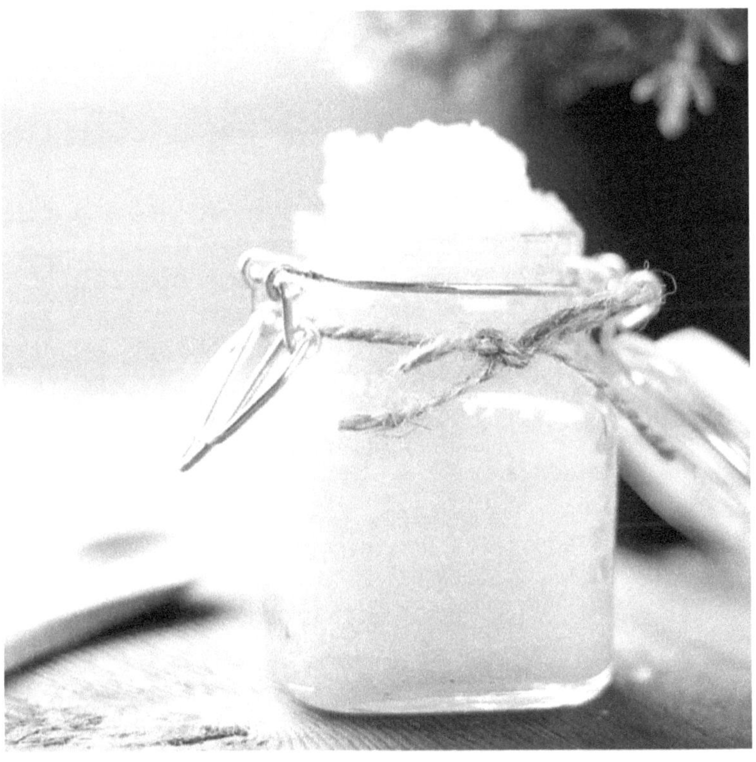

Lavender essential oil has antimicrobial properties which have profound benefits for your skin, especially acne- or spot-prone skin. It can also work wonders for acne scars, helping to reduce their appearance while promoting healing and rejuvenation.

Preparation Time: 10 mins

List of Ingredients:

- 1 cup white sugar
- ½ cup coconut oil
- 3 drops rosemary oil
- Scrapings of 1 vanilla bean
- 15 drops lavender oil

OOOOOOOOOOOOOOOOOOOOOOOOOOOOOOOOOOOOOOO

Procedure:

1. Combine all ingredients in a small bowl and mix well with a spoon.

2. Wet your clean face with warm water to make the scrub easier to massage into your skin.

3. Take a tablespoon of the scrub and gently rub it into your skin using small, circular motions. Rinse it off with warm water.

4. Soak a cotton pad in cold water and run it over your face to close your pores. Pat your face dry with a soft towel. Follow with a moisturizer after 30 minutes*.

5. Store any remaining scrub in a jar in the refrigerator.

*It's important to wait for your skin to calm a little before applying any further products.

(40) Green Tea and Aloe Scrub

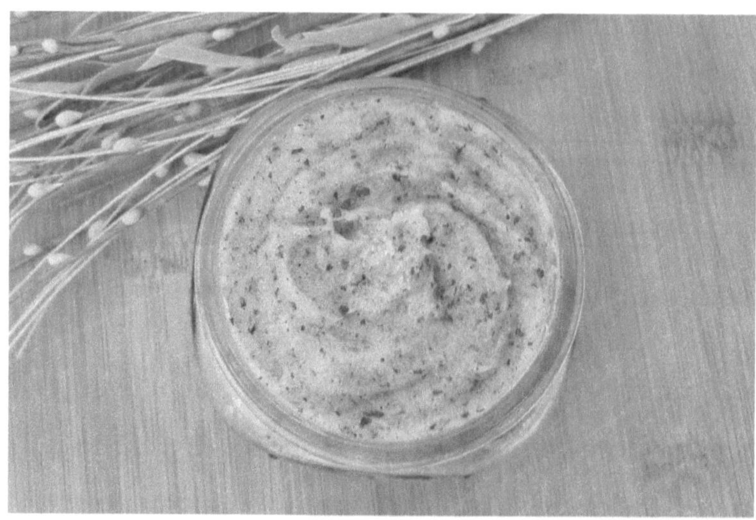

This great mask is perfect for acne-prone, oily skin. With the perfect balance of specific oils, this scrub with leave your face feeling soft, supple, and moisturized. It won't dry out your skin, so there is no need to use any lotion or moisturizing products after. Green tea will calm any current breakouts and tea tree oil will help to prevent any future ones. Win-win.

Preparation Time: 10 mins

List of Ingredients:

- ⅓ cup coconut oil
- ¼ cup sugar
- 1 tablespoon aloe vera jelly
- 2 organic green tea, tea bags
- 6 drops tea tree oil

ooooooooooooooooooooooooooooooooooooooo

Procedure:

1. Cut the top off both tea bags and add the contents to a small bowl. Add in all remaining ingredients and stir well to combined,

2. Apply a tablespoon of scrub to a clean, damp face and gently massage into the skin for 30-60 seconds. Rinse off with warm water, followed by cold. There is no need to moisturize with any other products after using this mask.

3. Store any remaining scrub in a jar in the refrigerator.*

* Scrub will last for 10-12 days in a refrigerator. Use no more than twice a week.

Author's Afterthoughts

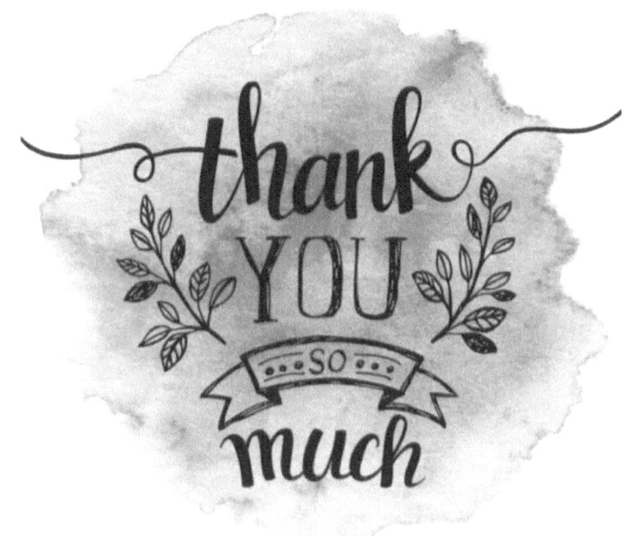

Thank you for reading my book. Your feedback is important to me. It would be greatly appreciated if you could please take a moment to REVIEW this book on Amazon so that we could make our next version better

Thanks!

Jenny Kings